Kratom for Beginners:

Eliminate Anxiety, Increase Focus & Live Happy With This Power of This Potent Plant

Table of Contents

Copyright

Introduction

Herbs have always been part of daily living. These can be sources of nutrition and flavoring. Herbs are also one of the main go-to remedy for aches and pains, health problems, and relief from stress. Some herbs can even help a person feel better, ease the mind and body, and improve energy levels. One such herb is kratom.

Find out what kratom is, what it can do and how to harness its benefits in the best and safest way. Read this book and find out:

- What is kratom

- Where is kratom found

- What are the different uses of kratom

- What are the available forms

- What are the different preparations

- How to prepare kratom to achieve the benefits

- What are the safe dosages

- What are the possible risks

- What are the precautions to follow

- What are the different safety guidelines

- And so much more

Read this book and get a deeper understanding of kratom.

Chapter 1 A Brief Glance at Kratom

Kratom is an indigenous tree to Southeast Asia. It is scientifically known as *Mitragyna speciosa Korthals*. Other names include *kakuam, thom* (southern regions of Thailand) and *ithang*. In Malaysia, the plant is known by the names *blak* or *ketum*. This tree abundantly grows in the villages of Thailand. It is also found in the northern portion of the Malay Peninsula extending toward Borneo.

It is considered a psychoactive plant, which contains several compounds that have benefits to the different organs of the body. For centuries, Thai villagers have been using katom as part of their daily life. They use it mainly to help improve their mood and motivation to face their daily tasks.

The Mitragyna speciosa

The tree grows to a full height of 15 meters or 50 feet. The canopy spreads over an area of about 4.5 meters or 15 feet. The flowers have yellow-colored petals. The leaves are glossy, dark green in color. The leaf shape is ovate-acuminate, which grow in opposite patterns along a stalk.

The tree is considered an evergreen instead of deciduous. It constantly sheds and replaces its leaves. More abundant leaf fall occurs during dry seasons. More vigorous new leaf growth occurs during rainy seasons. Cultivated trees in environmental conditions outside of the natural tropical conditions experience leaf fall at colder temperatures. Usually, leaves fall when the environmental temperatures drop to about 4 °C.

Seeds and Growth

Kratom trees grow from fresh seeds. These have low germination rates, ranging from 20 to 30%. Growth is best in wet soils that are rich in humus. The seedlings require large amounts of nutrients during the growing periods. Good growth requires rich and very fertile soils. The seedlings are also sensitive to drought conditions and frost, especially when grown outside of its native tropical habitat. Aside from seeds, kratom can be cultivated via cuttings, too.

There is very little information on how to cultivate kratom trees because both seeds and cuttings are difficult to find. Also, majority of those who have experience with kratom allow it to grow naturally without much interference. Commercial growers are just starting to experiment with cultivating the plant outside of its natural habitat. Another source of difficulty is rooting the cuttings. It is difficult for the cutting to establish enough root system for survival. But once they do, they are somewhat hardy. However, they can still be prone to fungal attacks that destroy their xylem. Many people are turning to cloning instead because of this difficulty.

Chapter 2 Uses and Effects of Kratom

There are many alkaloids present in kratom. The most active and responsible for most of kratom's effects is the alkaloid mitragynine. This is an opioid agonist, which means that mitragynine has a strong affinity with the brain's opioid receptors. Anxiety and mood regulation are affected by these same receptors. This capability allows mitragynine to exert influence over one's moods and level of anxiety.

When mitragynine binds with the brain's opioid receptors, it produces an improvement in the mood. It stimulates a feeling of euphoria, which is similar to the effects of opiates like opium and heroin. The difference between opiates and mitragynine is on the specific receptor sites. Opiates bind to *mu* receptors while mitragynine binds to *delta* receptors. When taken at high doses, mitragynine can also stimulate the *mu* receptors. This characteristic allows kratom to produce a stimulating effect when taken in low doses and produce narcotic effects when taken at high doses. Because of the difference in specific opiate receptors, there is much less risk for addiction with kratom use.

Understanding the effects

As has been mentioned, there are 2 basic effects from kratom use. The effects depend on the dose. The stimulant effect is achieved by taking low doses of kratom. During this time, a person experiences heightened alertness. The physical energy is increased, as well as sexual energy. There is also increased talkativeness with enhanced sociability and friendliness.

At higher doses, a person experiences the sedative-analgesic-euphoric levels. There is less sensitivity to both emotional and physical types of pain. There is calmness, with a general sense of comfort and pleasure. To some, this state produces a dream-like quality to reality. There is also increased appreciation for music. This is why most people who use kratom for recreational purposes tend to experience enhanced creative thinking.

In some people, there are reports of sweating and itching all over the body. Pupil constriction occurs. Nausea may be evident, which can easily be relieved with by lying down and relaxing.

There are reports that kratom can increase sexual desire or libido in women. Men also experience reduced problems with erection (either in achieving or in maintaining erection). These are believed to be caused by the decrease in anxiety levels that may be affecting sexual desire and energy.

There are also other effects from kratom use. There is a decrease in the tone of the smooth muscles. This means slowed heart rates and reduced blood pressure, as well as slower deeper respirations. It also produces a local anesthetic effect. Sometimes, kratom may also induce depression of the central nervous system functioning.

Kratom effects usually last for 6 hours. Higher doses will result to more potent effects that last longer. Also, most people who took kratom report feeling a positive afterglow, which can often last well in the following day. The effects start to manifest after 5-10 minutes of intake.

Specific Uses

There are many uses for kratom, although, these uses still need more research for verification. Most of these are based mainly on user reports and on a small number of limited studies.

Stimulant

This is the traditional use of kratom. Peasants, farmers and laborers in Thailand commonly use kratom for this its stimulant effect. They used it as a means to relax their mind and bodies after a hard day's work. They also use this as a means to cope with the stresses (mental, emotional and physical) of daily living. A number of villagers use kratom every day. There are some studies conducted that found no problems with addiction despite the daily use.

Villagers would chew kratom leaves about 3 to 10 times a day. New users chew only a few leaves. Long term users chew as much as 30 leaves per day. Some also may need to gradually increase leaf-chewing the longer they use kratom. This gradual need to increase the amount of intake may stem from the development of tolerance.

Aside from using kratom to help them get through the day, villagers also use it to help them with work. They use kratom to enhance their energy. This can help them to work harder and accomplish more from the day's work. Some also report enhanced motivation after taking kratom, giving them a stronger desire to work.

Mood Regulation and Anxiety Reduction

One of the main reasons for the use of kratom is its ability to regulate one's mood and reduce levels of anxiety. Mood and anxiety are regulated by the brain through the neurotransmitters. Most modern-day medications for mood and anxiety problems affect the levels of serotonin. This neurotransmitter is known to improve mood and decreases anxiety levels when its levels are increased. However, the improvement is relatively mild and does not last long. When opiate receptors, as well as dopamine levels are stimulated, the improvements in anxiety and mood are more profound. The reason for this is because serotonin has a mild and non-addictive effect to the body. Opiates and dopamine produce stronger effects. However, these can be highly addictive. Mitragynine in kratom stimulates the opiate receptors but is in itself non-addictive compared to opiates. It has a more profound effect on mood and anxiety, minus the addiction.

ADD (Attention Deficit Disorder in Adults)

There are some reports that claim kratom can help in managing the symptoms of ADD or attention deficit disorder in adults. However, this still needs more scientific evidence. The belief is based on the mood-enhancing effect of kratom. This can help manage some of the ADD symptoms such as hyperactivity and emotional problems like frustration, mood swings and irritability and decreased motivation. Because mitragynine in kratom also enhances focus, it helps manage other ADD symptoms such as difficulty focusing and staying with tasks, procrastination and decreased productivity.

Substitute for opium

Opium is a highly addictive substance. Kratom can be used to gradually wean off a person from opium addiction. In a few days, the person would be able to stop the addictive use of narcotics such as opium. Cravings for the addictive substance are reduced, as well as the intensity of the withdrawal symptoms. Kratom for treatment of opium addiction is common in East Asia.

In New Zealand, kratom is used as part of the detoxification process for methadone addiction. Patients are given kratom, which they smoke whenever they feel any withdrawal symptom. This kind of treatment is given for 6 weeks. There is moderate success rate for this kratom treatment, with patients report experiencing visualization effects (i.e., vivid dreams) at night.

Recreation

Recently, more and more people use kratom for recreational purposes. It is gaining popularity because of the narcotic-like state it induces at high doses. It stimulates euphoria, which is similar to that induced by heroin. However, this effect is not as profound as the state one achieves with heroin. Some believe that kratom is a safer alternative to recreational drugs such as heroin and marijuana because it is not as addictive.

Some users report that even with the sense of euphoria, they still feel they have enough energy to function well for the day. This is unlike heroin and other recreational drugs where one can no longer perform normal daily activities.

Kratom Strains and their specific effects

Kratom is used in different ways and the effects also differ. The different strains come from Bali, Thailand, and Malaysia. The differences in the effects are attributed to the genetic differences, which causes the production of different alkaloids and indoles.

Bali strain

The Bali strain (from Indonesia) reportedly stimulates narcosis and relaxation when taken at higher doses. At lower doses, this strain produces a stimulant effect.

Malaysian strain

Kratom from Malaysia has an almost identical effect to the Bali strain.

Thai strain

The effects of the Thai strain reportedly lasts longer, compared to other strains. It also produces the most sedative effects. This strain is also one of the most widely commercially available strains. This strain is also no longer confined to growing in Thailand. Other countries are also cultivating the Thai strain for commercial uses. The recommended normal dose for Thai kratom is around 3 to 5 grams.

Maeng Da

Maeng Da is another strain originating from Thailand. The literal translation is "pimp grade". This is the strongest, most potent strain currently available in the market. It produces less euphoria compared to other strains but produces more energizing effects. Some critics claim that Maeng Da kratom effects are more of jitteriness than energizing and that the effects do not last long. Active dose is at 1 to 2 grams. The color of high quality Maeng Da is deep, bright green.

Chapter 3 How to Use Kratom

There are many ways to prepare and take kratom to harness its benefits.

Available forms

There are several types of kratom commercially available today. This includes the tea form, powder form, capsule, resin and whole leaves. Powder and resin forms are reportedly more potent than the leaves. The potency of any of these types and formulations depend on the quality and age of the plant source. "Commercial kratom leaves" refers to a blend of leaves of different qualities, which means the high quality ones are mixed with poor ones.

Dosage

The dosage depends on the form and quality of kratom. Using higher quality kratom would require lower dosages.

Generally, for new users, 5 to 10 grams is recommended when using dried leaves. If using the powdered form, use lower dosages because it is stronger than whole leaves. Use only 3 to 5 grams. When using the resin form, use also in lower dosages, at 3 to 5 grams.

Again, kratom use is not habit-forming, as long as it is used properly and responsibly. Also, use kratom only 1-2 times per month. Regular users should expect the need to increase dosage to obtain the same level of effect after prolonged use.

Preparations

Leaves

The traditional way of taking kratom is by chewing fresh leaves after the central, stringy vein is removed. Some chew the dried leaves, too. Warm water or tea is drank after chewing the leaves to wash it all down. Some crush the dried leaves and turn them into tea or powder form for easy swallowing.

Tea

To make kratom tea, place powdered kratom leaves in a cup of hot water, about 5 to 10 grams. Let the powdered leaves steep in the water for 10 to 15 minutes. Or, get the same amount of dried leaves (5-10grams) and crush these into smaller bits, Steep in a cup of hot water. After 5 to 10 minutes, the tea is strained and then drunk. This method is most common among users in the West. Some mix kratom tea with black or other herbal teas to improve the taste. Some add honey or sugar as sweeteners.

Paste

Another way to use kratom leaves is by producing a paste-like extract. The dried or fresh leaves are boiled for long hours to release the extract. The leaves are then discarded and the extract is made into small pellets. Extracts are stored, which can be used at a later time. The mall pellets are swallowed much like tablets or pills. Some dissolve the extract pellets in hot water and drink it as tea.

Powdered kratom

This preparation is actually finely crushed dried kratom leaves. Powdered kratom can be mixed with applesauce or fruit juices for easy swallowing. This combination also masks the taste, which some people may not find very attractive.

Smoking kratom

Some people smoke kratom. However, this form of intake has no significant advantage over taking kratom as tea or chewing leaves. Also, when smoking kratom, a huge amount of leaves would have to be smoked just to get the recommended dosages.

Capsules

The most convenient way to take kratom without having to deal with the unpleasantly bitter taste is with capsules. Some people choose to make their own kratom capsules to make sure that only high quality leaves are used and that no other compounds are mixed in.

Leaves should be finely ground before placing in capsules. Use a precision scale that weighs accurately up to the milligrams when measuring the contents for each capsule. This will ensure that each capsule delivers constant and accurate amounts of kratom. Weigh the same dosage as mentioned in previous section (5 to 10 grams). Use capsules that come in size "00". It may be difficult to place the contents into small capsules, so a capsule maker may come in handy.

If making capsules for personal use is not an option, there are commercially available kratom capsules. Make sure to get from credible sources.

Dosages for kratom capsules also vary, depending on kratom strain, age of the plant source and quality of the leaves used. Generally, the following guidelines can be used:

- To get mild kratom effects, take 1 to 4 capsules or 2 to 6 grams. The effect is typically stimulant, evidenced by more focus and better energy levels.

- To get medium level of kratom effects, take 5 to 7 capsules or 7 to 15 grams. The effects are typically stimulant-like. Some describe this level of effect as sedative-analgesic-euphoric.

- To get the strong levels of kratom effects, take 8 to 10 capsules, about 16 to 25v grams. The effects are more on analgesic, euphoric and sedative. This dosage is most often too strong for new users and for people who are highly sensitive to the alkaloids present in kratom.

- Some people, particularly long-term users may take higher doses, at 26 to 50 grams. The effects are already very potent, producing analgesic, sedative and euphoric sensations. For most people, this is extremely potent and generally unsafe.

It is recommended to take a maximum of 10 capsules and no more for safety. This is especially so for those who are new to kratom. However, taking more capsules may be acceptable for regular users who have already developed tolerance (no longer gets the desired effects with previous lower doses).

Dosage guidelines are based on the amount of kratom leaves and not extracts. This is applicable for those chewing fresh or dried leaves and for those taking teas. Extracts have different concentrations of kratom alkaloids.

Sensitivity to kratom effects varies among different people. Some achieve mild effects with higher doses. Some strong effects with low doses. These dosage guidelines are just loose approximations. Individuals should check for their reactions before they decide on the appropriate dose for their needs.

It is also most recommended to start with low doses. Wait for a minimum of 3 hours after kratom intake to experience the effects. If the level reached is not the desired one, take a slightly higher dose the next time. However, do not take doses one after another. That is, wait a few days before adjusting the doses. For example, take 4 capsules in the morning and wait 3 hours for the effects to become evident. If the level of the effect is not the one desired, take the next higher dose after a few days, not immediately within the same day.

Liquid extracts that resemble tea is also a growing popular way of preparing kratom leaves. The basic recipe is as follows:

- Measure 50 grams of kratom leaves, dried and crushed. Place these in a pot and add a liter of clean, drinking water.

- Boil the water with the leaves over medium high heat for about 15 to 20 minutes.

- After the mixture boils, remove from heat. Pour and strain into a large bowl. Reserve and set aside this liquid.

- Take the leaves in the strainer. Squeeze all remaining liquid and add it to the rest of the liquid in the bowl.

- Take the strained leaves and place them back into the pot. Get 1 more liter of water and add it to the pot. Boil this again for 15 to 20 minutes and repeat the rest of the process 2 more times.

- After the last boiling, discard the leaves.

- Combine the liquid from all the boiling and place them all back in the same pot. Boil the combined liquids under medium high heat until the volume is reduced to 100 ml.

This preparation can be stored safely in the refrigerator and will keep for 5 days. Adding a small amount of alcohol can help make this preparation keep longer. Adding 10% alcohol will extend the extract's storage life for months, as long as it is keep in the refrigerator. To get the 10%, add 1 part alcohol (e.g., vodka, rum, whisky, etc.) to 3 parts of liquid tea-like kratom extract.

Chapter 4 Side Effects and Precautions

Kratom is a herbal preparation that has long been used by a lot of people. While a small number of studies and observations have found that kratom is safe to use, there are still safety guidelines and precautions to consider to ensure full benefits with minimum risk.

Risks

Kratom is generally safe, especially if using high quality leaves, used properly in the right doses and not combined with other drugs, supplements or herbs. The effects range from mild to strong depending on the dosage.

The greatest risk is when users perform hazardous activities such as operating heavy or sensitive machineries, using power tools, and driving while under kratom effects. Also, avoid climbing ladders or working at heights. The sedating effects may reduce decision-making skills. Avoid these activities while experiencing kratom effects, even at mild levels. Also, avoid any activities that require critical focus to avoid any untoward incident.

Also, refrain from doing activities requiring close and constant attention. Even at low doses, kratom can make a person fall asleep. Do not bake or cook while under kratom effects. Leaving the stove or oven on and then fall asleep may cause fire.

The best way to reduce risks is to use kratom during relaxation times. Use these when there aren't any crucial tasks to perform.

Also, never take kratom when pregnant or planning to get pregnant. Safety has not yet been established for the pregnant woman and her baby. Also, never use when breastfeeding as some of the alkaloids may be excreted in the breast milk. Safety is also not established for newborns, babies and children.

Is kratom habit-forming or addictive?

Although there isn't any sufficient studies made, observations have shown that kratom is not likely to cause habit or addiction. However, some people do become dependent on kratom, as observed among the villagers in Thailand. When used responsibly, kratom do not cause addiction or dependence. Even among recreational users, kratom poses virtually zero risk for addiction.

Taking kratom on a daily basis can become a habit, though. It is much like caffeine or tobacco use. Daily intake can produce a habit, but not an addiction. Some daily users feel they need to take kratom to help get through the day. This is very similar in some people who need to take coffee to help them keep focused or get them energized. Some people are more prone to develop habits than others. Once it becomes difficult to stay within the safety guidelines of kratom use, immediately quit using. For example, safety guidelines recommend kratom use to 1-2 times in a month only, maximum of one dose in a week. If there is a craving or feeling of needing to take more often, stop kratom use immediately.

Precautions and Safety Guidelines

Precautions need to be exercised to achieve the best results under the safest conditions. Kratom may be plant-based but the alkaloids still have the potential to produce negative side effects.

For safety and for best results, follow these guidelines:

- Never take high doses when using kratom for the first few times or when changing preparations.

- Adjust dosages gradually to achieve desired effects.

- New users should stay with doses below 10 grams to avoid discomforts such as nausea.

- Avoid taking more than 25 grams to prevent nausea and other discomforts.

- Take kratom on an empty stomach when taking high doses.

- Strong doses may produce adverse reactions such as prolonged and severe vomiting episodes in hypersensitive people.

- Use kratom as an occasional treat and never on a daily basis. Too frequent use leads to less pleasurable gains. This also increases the possibility of kratom use becoming a habit that can be difficult to break.

Side Effects

So far, from observations of Thai villagers who have been using it for a long time, kratom is safe. It does not produce any health problems as long as it is not used too frequently and in large quantities.

Daily kratom use isn't generally recommended, but there are a few people in Thailand who do. It has been observed that people who can tolerate daily use develop dark pigmentations on their faces, as well as weight loss. Physical symptoms of withdrawal are also observed when they do not take their daily dose of kratom. Withdrawal symptoms include the following:

- Runny nose
- Crying or increased lacrimation
- Diarrhea
- Irritability
- Muscle aches
- Jerky movements of the muscles

Just like any other drug or herb, kratom can produce negative reactions to insensitive individuals. There is also the possibility for allergic reactions depending on the person's overall health and tendencies. Also, negative or any untoward or unusual reactions may be a result of poor quality plant source or poor preparation.

Drug-Herb/Herb Drug Combination

Some people combine several herbs with kratom. This is generally not recommended, although some practice this and do not experience any negative effects. There were also reports of pleasant effects without any negative or unwanted side effects. Adding ordinary tea is safe, though.

Some choose to combine kratom tea with other herbal teas that have sedative, narcotic and/or euphoric effects. Others add tea from red flowers from the poppy plant, *Papaver rhoeas*. This plant produces an extremely mild narcotic effect. Some also combine kratom tea with blue lotus tea. The blue lotus tea is made from the blue lotus plant, *Nymphaea caerulea*, which produces sedation and euphoria when ingested.

Generally, mixing herbs that produce the same or opposing effects are not recommended. The effects are often unpredictable. The combination may either produce very high levels or may cancel each other's effects.

Also, adding alcohol in small quantities is safe. But do not take them separately. That is, do not drink kratom and then follow it up with alcohol. Adding alcohol is just to prolong the storage life of kratom tea preparations. However, never go beyond the 10% alcohol (1part alcohol to 3 parts kratom tea) concentration.

Some combinations may produce serious negative effects because of certain reactions. Do not take kratom together with the following:

- Caffeine, in large doses
- Cocaine
- Yohimbine
- Amphetamine and similar substances

Kratom in combination with these substances may over-stimulate the body and increase the blood pressure.

Do not take kratom when taking any MAOI drug, *Banesteriosis caapi*, and Syrian rue. This combination may lead to serious or fatal adverse reactions.

Conclusion

Thank you for purchasing this book.

I hope that you were able to learn more about kratom. This herb can help produce a pleasant, relaxing and at the same time, stimulating effect in the body. Caution should always be exercised, as you should with all drugs, supplements and herbs. Also, it is very important to be aware of how your body reacts to kratom. If you experience any discomfort, stop. Also, always consult your doctor before taking kratom and before you take anything while on kratom. If you have any health problems, it is best not to take kratom, especially if you have problems with the cardiovascular system or you have history with stroke, diabetes, and allergies.

Remember, kratom is supposed to help you feel better. To get the maximum benefits, be a responsible user.

Again, thank you.